KRISTA JAMES

Easy Essential Oil Recipes

What else can you do with essential oils aside from diffusing? Make cookies, lip balm, bug spray, soaps and more!

Contents

1

Introduction

Here it is! The Easy Essential Oil Recipe Book – your new best friend in all things aromatic and fun! Get ready to dive into a world beyond just diffusing, where we'll whip up fantastic creations together. Let's find out what else you can do with your oils aside from diffusing them!

Picture this: Lavender Mint Soaps that make your shower feel like a spa, Peppermint Chocolate Chip Cookies that are basically happiness in each bite, and Lip Balms so good, you'll wonder how you ever lived without them!

But it's not just about indulging your sweet tooth or pampering your skin. We've got tricks up our sleeves to keep those annoying bugs at bay with our homemade repellents. And for those days when you need a little extra TLC, there are foot soaks, room sprays, and stress-relief rollers – all infused with the magic of essential oils.

No complicated stuff here! Just easy, breezy recipes that'll make you feel like an essential oil pro in no time. So, grab your oils, join the party, and let's make every day a little more fabulous!

2

Safety First

Alright, let's talk safety before we jump into these easy essential oil recipes. Here's the lowdown on keeping things safe and enjoyable. And, if you're gifting these creations, don't forget to pass along the safety info!

General Guidelines

Patch Test: Always conduct a patch test before using any new essential oil, especially if you have sensitive skin or are prone to allergies. Apply a small amount of the diluted mixture to a small area and wait 24 hours to check for any adverse reactions.

Dilution: Essential oils are potent, and proper dilution is key. Follow recommended dilution ratios in each recipe to avoid skin irritation or sensitization.

Pregnancy and Medical Conditions: If you are pregnant, nursing, or have underlying health conditions or concerns, consult with a healthcare professional before using essential oils. Some oils may not be suitable during pregnancy or for certain medical conditions.

Quality: For recipes involving ingestion, such as lip balms or cookies, ensure you use high-quality essential oils labeled as food-grade. Not all essential oils are suitable for consumption, so choose wisely to enhance both safety and flavor. Consult with a healthcare professional if you have concerns or specific health conditions.

3

Soap Recipes

Okay, it's time! Let the fun begin and enjoy these easy essential oil recipes! What's better than having clean hands? Having clean hands that smell like your favorite essential oils! Mm mm mm....

3.1 Lavender Mint Soap

Ingredients

- 1 cup melt-and-pour soap base
- 10 drops lavender essential oil
- 5 drops peppermint essential oil

Instructions

1. Melt the soap base according to package instructions.
2. Stir in the essential oils (mix well).
3. Pour the mixture into soap molds and let it cool and harden.

Shopping List

- Melt-and-pour soap base
- Lavender essential oil
- Peppermint essential oil
- Soap molds

Essential Oil Information

Lavender Essential Oil

- Description: Lavender oil is known for its calming and soothing aroma. It has floral and herbaceous notes.
- Common Uses: Lavender oil is often used to promote relaxation, alleviate stress, and support sleep.
- Warnings: Avoid direct contact with eyes and mouth. Perform a patch test before applying to the skin.

Peppermint Essential Oil

- Description: Peppermint oil has a refreshing and invigorating scent with a hint of menthol.
- Common Uses: Peppermint oil is popular for promoting mental clarity, easing headaches, and providing a cooling sensation.
- Warnings: Dilute properly before skin application. Avoid contact with eyes, nose, and sensitive areas.

3.2 Citrus Burst Soap

Ingredients

- 1 cup glycerin soap base
- 15 drops orange essential oil
- 10 drops lemon essential oil

Instructions

1. Melt the glycerin soap base.
2. Mix in the essential oils (mix well).
3. Pour the mixture into molds and let it set.

Shopping List

- Glycerin soap base
- Orange essential oil
- Lemon essential oil
- Soap molds

Essential Oil Information

Orange Essential Oil

- Description: Orange oil carries a bright and uplifting citrus fragrance.
- Common Uses: Often used to boost mood, reduce stress, and add a fresh scent to environments.
- Warnings: Citrus oils can cause photosensitivity. Avoid exposure to direct sunlight after application.

Lemon Essential Oil

- Description: Lemon oil has a zesty and invigorating scent.
- Common Uses: Known for its refreshing aroma, lemon oil is often used for energizing and purifying spaces.
- Warnings: Dilute properly before skin application. Avoid contact with eyes and sunlight after use.

3.3 Tea Tree & Eucalyptus Antibacterial Soap

Ingredients

- 1 cup shea butter soap base
- 10 drops tea tree essential oil
- 10 drops eucalyptus essential oil

Instructions

1. Melt the shea butter soap base.
2. Add the essential oils and mix thoroughly.
3. Pour the mixture into molds and allow it to solidify.

Shopping List

- Shea butter soap base
- Tea tree essential oil
- Eucalyptus essential oil
- Soap molds

Essential Oil Information

Tea Tree Essential Oil

- Description: Tea tree oil possesses a fresh and medicinal aroma.
- Common Uses: Known for its antibacterial properties, tea tree oil is often used in skincare and cleaning products.
- Warnings: Can cause skin irritation in some individuals. Perform a patch test before widespread use.

Eucalyptus Essential Oil

- Description: Eucalyptus oil has a camphor and invigorating scent.
- Common Uses: Often used to promote respiratory health and as a natural antibacterial agent.
- Warnings: Use with caution, as excessive use may cause skin irritation. Avoid contact with eyes and sensitive areas.

3.4 Rosemary and Peppermint Energizing Soap

Ingredients

- 1 cup goat milk soap base
- 10 drops rosemary essential oil
- 8 drops peppermint essential oil

Instructions

1. Melt the goat milk soap base.
2. Stir in the essential oils until thoroughly combined.
3. Pour the mixture into molds and allow it to cool.

Shopping List

- Goat milk soap base
- Rosemary essential oil
- Peppermint essential oil
- Soap molds

Essential Oil Information

Rosemary Essential Oil

- Description: Rosemary oil has a fresh, herbaceous scent.
- Common Uses: Known for promoting focus and energy, rosemary oil is often used in aromatherapy.
- Warnings: Avoid during pregnancy and in individuals with certain medical conditions including epilepsy.

Peppermint Essential Oil

- Description: Peppermint oil carries a cool and invigorating aroma.
- Common Uses: Widely used for its refreshing properties, peppermint oil is known to enhance mental alertness.
- Warnings: Dilute properly, as it can be irritating to the skin. Avoid contact with eyes and sensitive areas.

3.5 Calming Chamomile Soap

Ingredients

- 1 cup olive oil soap base
- 12 drops chamomile essential oil

Instructions

1. Melt the olive oil soap base.
2. Add the chamomile essential oil and mix thoroughly.
3. Pour the mixture into molds and allow it to set.

Shopping List

- Olive oil soap base
- Chamomile essential oil
- Soap molds

Essential Oil Information

Chamomile Essential Oil

- Description: Chamomile oil has a sweet and calming fragrance.
- Common Uses: Renowned for its relaxing properties, chamomile oil is often used to promote a sense of calm and tranquility.
- Warnings: Avoid during pregnancy and if allergic to plants in the Asteraceae family.

4

Lip Balm Recipes

If you're as crazy about lip balms as you are about essential oils, get ready to have a blast making all of these! And don't forget to try the Chocolate Mint Lip Scrub in the Body Scrub section!

4.1 Vanilla Honey Lip Balm

Ingredients

- 2 tbsp coconut oil
- 1 tbsp beeswax
- 1 tsp honey
- 5 drops vanilla essential oil

Instructions

1. Melt the coconut oil and beeswax together.
2. Stir in the honey and vanilla essential oil (mix well).
3. Pour the mixture into lip balm containers to cool.

Shopping List

- Coconut oil
- Beeswax
- Honey
- Vanilla essential oil
- Lip balm containers

Essential Oil Information

Vanilla Essential Oil

- Description: Vanilla oil has a sweet, comforting aroma reminiscent of freshly baked goods.
- Common Uses: Often used for its soothing and relaxing properties, vanilla oil can add a delightful fragrance to various recipes.
- Warnings: None known.

4.2 Peppermint Cocoa Lip Balm

Ingredients

- 2 tbsp cocoa butter
- 1 tbsp coconut oil
- 10 drops peppermint essential oil

Instructions

1. Melt the cocoa butter and coconut oil.
2. Add the peppermint essential oil and mix well.
3. Pour the mixture into lip balm tubes and allow it to solidify.

Shopping List

- Cocoa butter
- Coconut oil
- Peppermint essential oil
- Lip balm tubes

Essential Oil Information

Peppermint Essential Oil

- Description: Peppermint oil boasts a refreshing and invigorating scent with a cool, minty undertone.
- Common Uses: Known for its energizing properties, peppermint oil can uplift the senses and add a pleasant aroma to cosmetic recipes.
- Warnings: Avoid using peppermint oil on or near the face of infants and young children.

4.3 Citrus Bliss Lip Balm

Ingredients

- 2 tbsp shea butter
- 1 tbsp sweet almond oil
- 10 drops citrus essential oil blend

Instructions

1. Melt the shea butter and sweet almond oil.
2. Stir in the citrus essential oil blend (mix well).
3. Pour the mixture into lip balm containers and let it set.

Shopping List

- Shea butter
- Sweet almond oil
- Citrus essential oil blend
- Lip balm containers

Essential Oil Information

Citrus Essential Oil Blend

- Description: A harmonious blend of citrus oils, providing a vibrant and uplifting aroma.
- Common Uses: Citrus essential oil blends are known for their refreshing scent, promoting a positive atmosphere.
- Warnings: Some citrus oils can cause photosensitivity, so avoid exposure to direct sunlight after application.

4.4 Lavender Mint Lip Balm

Ingredients

- 2 tbsp beeswax
- 1 tbsp coconut oil
- 8 drops lavender essential oil
- 5 drops peppermint essential oil

Instructions

1. Melt the beeswax and coconut oil.
2. Mix in the lavender and peppermint oils (mix well).
3. Pour the mixture into lip balm containers and let it set.

Shopping List

- Beeswax
- Coconut oil
- Lavender essential oil
- Peppermint essential oil
- Lip balm containers

Essential Oil Information

Lavender Essential Oil

- Description: Lavender oil offers a floral and calming aroma, promoting relaxation.
- Common Uses: Known for its soothing properties, lavender oil is often used for relaxation and skincare.

- Warnings: Lavender oil is generally safe, but it's advisable to conduct a patch test, especially for individuals with sensitive skin.

Peppermint Essential Oil

- Description: Peppermint oil provides a cool and invigorating scent, revitalizing the senses.
- Common Uses: Peppermint oil is popular for its refreshing qualities, often used for alertness and respiratory support.
- Warnings: Avoid using peppermint oil on or near the face of infants and young children, as it may cause respiratory distress.

4.5 Coconut Lime Lip Balm

Ingredients

- 2 tbsp coconut oil
- 1 tbsp beeswax
- 1 tsp lime essential oil

Instructions

1. Begin by gathering the following ingredients for your Coconut Lime Lip Balm.
2. In a heat-resistant container, melt 2 tbsp of coconut oil and 1 tbsp of beeswax using a double boiler or microwave.
3. Once melted, stir in 1 tsp of lime essential oil, ensuring an even distribution of the fragrance.
4. Carefully pour the infused mixture into lip balm containers, making

it easy to apply.

5. Allow the lip balm to cool and solidify, providing a smooth consistency for use.

Shopping List

- Coconut oil
- Beeswax
- Lime essential oil
- Lip balm containers

Essential Oil Information

Lime Essential Oil

- Description: Lime essential oil, extracted from Citrus aurantiifolia, presents a lively and citrusy aroma. Recognized for its invigorating properties, it brings a refreshing touch to beauty and self-care products.
- Common Uses: Lip Balm: Elevate lip care with the Coconut Lime Lip Balm, delivering a delightful citrus experience. Skin Care: Dilute and apply topically for potential skin benefits.
- Warnings: Skin Sensitivity: Conduct a patch test before applying directly to the skin. Photosensitivity: Avoid direct sunlight exposure after applying to the skin, as citrus oils may cause photosensitivity. Dilution: Dilute appropriately before topical application.

5

Bug Repellent Recipes

Not sure about you, but bugs LOVE me and I hate them. Bug repellent is a must, but natural recipes are the only way to go.

5.1 Citronella and Lemongrass Bug Spray

Ingredients

- 2 oz distilled water
- 2 oz witch hazel
- 20 drops citronella essential oil
- 10 drops lemongrass essential oil

Instructions

1. Mix the distilled water and witch hazel in a small glass spray bottle.
2. Add citronella and lemongrass oils.
3. Shake well before use.

Shopping List

- Distilled water
- Witch hazel
- Citronella essential oil
- Lemongrass essential oil
- Small glass spray bottle

Essential Oil Information

Citronella Essential Oil

- Description: Citronella oil has a fresh, citrusy scent that is commonly associated with repelling insects.
- Common Uses: It is widely used in insect repellent products and is known for its bug-repelling properties.
- Warnings: Citronella oil is generally safe but should be used with caution in high concentrations.

Lemongrass Essential Oil

- Description: Lemongrass oil has a bright and citrusy aroma, often used for its refreshing and uplifting qualities.
- Common Uses: Known for its insect-repelling properties, lemongrass oil is commonly used in bug sprays.
- Warnings: Lemongrass oil is considered safe for most people when used topically but may cause skin irritation in some individuals. Always conduct a patch test.

5.2 Eucalyptus and Tea Tree Anti-Mosquito Spray

Ingredients

- 2 oz distilled water
- 2 oz aloe vera gel
- 15 drops eucalyptus essential oil
- 10 drops tea tree essential oil

Instructions

1. Combine the distilled water and aloe vera gel in a small glass spray bottle.
2. Add eucalyptus and tea tree oils and mix well.

Shopping List

- Distilled water
- Aloe vera gel
- Eucalyptus essential oil
- Tea tree essential oil
- Small glass spray bottle

Essential Oil Information

Eucalyptus Essential Oil

- Description: Eucalyptus oil has a fresh and camphor scent, known for its invigorating and respiratory-supporting properties.
- Common Uses: It is often used in aromatherapy for its refreshing aroma and is a common ingredient in insect repellents.

- Warnings: Eucalyptus oil should be used with caution around young children, and it can cause skin irritation in some individuals.

Tea Tree Essential Oil

- Description: Tea tree oil has a medicinal and herbaceous scent, renowned for its antibacterial and antifungal properties.
- Common Uses: It is commonly used for skin issues and is an ingredient in natural insect repellents.
- Warnings: Tea tree oil is generally safe when used topically but may cause skin irritation in some individuals. Always conduct a patch test.

5.3 Lavender and Peppermint Bug Repellent

Ingredients

- 2 oz fractionated coconut oil
- 15 drops lavender essential oil
- 10 drops peppermint essential oil

Instructions

1. Mix fractionated coconut oil with lavender and peppermint essential oils in a small glass spray bottle.
2. Apply the mixture to exposed skin before heading outdoors.

Shopping List

- Fractionated coconut oil
- Lavender essential oil
- Peppermint essential oil
- Small glass spray bottle

Essential Oil Information

Lavender Essential Oil

- Description: Lavender oil has a sweet, floral aroma known for its calming and soothing properties.
- Common Uses: It is widely used for relaxation and may help repel insects naturally.
- Warnings: Lavender oil is generally safe but may cause skin irritation in some individuals. Always conduct a patch test.

Peppermint Essential Oil

- Description: Peppermint oil has a refreshing and minty scent, known for its invigorating and cooling effects.
- Common Uses: It is commonly used to deter pests and has a refreshing aroma.
- Warnings: Peppermint oil should be used with caution around young children, and it can cause skin irritation in some individuals. Conduct a patch test before use.

5.4 Rosemary Citrus Tick Repellent

Ingredients

- 2 oz almond oil
- 15 drops rosemary essential oil
- 10 drops citrus essential oil blend

Instructions

1. Combine almond oil with rosemary and citrus essential oils in a small glass spray bottle.
2. Apply to skin, avoiding the face.

Shopping List

- Almond oil
- Rosemary essential oil
- Citrus essential oil blend
- Small glass spray bottle

Essential Oil Information

Rosemary Essential Oil

- Description: Rosemary oil has a fresh, herbaceous aroma known for its invigorating and stimulating properties.
- Common Uses: It is often used as a natural insect repellent and for its refreshing scent.
- Warnings: Rosemary oil is generally safe but should be avoided during pregnancy and by individuals with epilepsy.

Citrus Essential Oil Blend

- Description: A blend of citrus oils with a bright and uplifting fragrance.
- Common Uses: Known for its refreshing and mood-boosting properties.
- Warnings: Citrus oils can cause skin sensitivity in some individuals. Avoid exposure to sunlight after application. Conduct a patch test before use.

5.5 Cedarwood and Geranium Fly Repellent

Ingredients

- 2 oz apple cider vinegar
- 15 drops cedarwood essential oil
- 10 drops geranium essential oil

Instructions

1. Mix apple cider vinegar with cedarwood and geranium essential oils in a small glass spray bottle.
2. Use a cloth to apply the mixture on exposed skin.

Shopping List

- Apple cider vinegar
- Cedarwood essential oil
- Geranium essential oil

- Small glass spray bottle

Essential Oil Information

Cedarwood Essential Oil

- Description: Cedarwood oil has a warm, woody aroma and is known for its grounding and calming properties.
- Common Uses: Often used in insect repellents and for its soothing effects.
- Warnings: Cedarwood oil is generally safe but should be avoided during pregnancy.

Geranium Essential Oil

- Description: Geranium oil has a floral and slightly sweet aroma, known for its balancing and uplifting properties.
- Common Uses: Used in skincare and as an insect repellent.
- Warnings: Geranium oil is generally safe but may cause skin irritation in some individuals. Conduct a patch test before use.

5.6 Basic Bug Spray

Ingredients

- 2 ounces of witch hazel or vodka
- 2 ounces of distilled water
- 10 drops of citronella essential oil
- 10 drops of eucalyptus essential oil

- 10 drops of lavender essential oil
- 5 drops of peppermint essential oil
- 5 drops of tea tree essential oil

Instructions

1. In a glass spray bottle, combine witch hazel or vodka with distilled water. The alcohol in vodka can help preserve the spray.
2. Add the citronella, eucalyptus, lavender, peppermint, and tea tree essential oils to the mixture.
3. Close the bottle tightly and shake well to ensure that the essential oils are thoroughly mixed with the liquid.
4. Allow the bug spray to sit for at least 30 minutes before using to let the oils blend.
5. Store the bug spray in a cool, dark place when not in use.

Shopping List

- Witch hazel or vodka
- Distilled water
- Citronella essential oil
- Eucalyptus essential oil
- Lavender essential oil
- Peppermint essential oil
- Tea tree essential oil
- Glass spray bottle

Essential Oil Information

Citronella Essential Oil

- Description: Known for its strong, lemon-like aroma, citronella is commonly used to ward off insects.
- Common Uses: Commonly used as a natural insect repellent, citronella oil is also employed in aromatherapy for mood enhancement and in cleaning products for its antibacterial qualities.
- Warnings: Caution is advised for skin sensitivity, potential phototoxicity, and allergies, and pregnant individuals should consult with a healthcare professional before using citronella essential oil.

Eucalyptus Essential Oil

- Description: Eucalyptus oil has a fresh and camphor scent, known for its invigorating and respiratory-supporting properties.
- Common Uses: It is often used in aromatherapy for its refreshing aroma and is a common ingredient in insect repellents.
- Warnings: Eucalyptus oil should be used with caution around young children, and it can cause skin irritation in some individuals.

Lavender Essential Oil

- Description: Lavender oil has a sweet, floral aroma known for its calming and soothing properties.
- Common Uses: It is widely used for relaxation and may help repel insects naturally.
- Warnings: Lavender oil is generally safe but may cause skin irritation in some individuals. Always conduct a patch test.

Peppermint Essential Oil

- Description: Peppermint oil has a refreshing and minty scent, known for its invigorating and cooling effects.
- Common Uses: It is commonly used to deter pests and has a refreshing aroma.
- Warnings: Peppermint oil should be used with caution around young children, and it can cause skin irritation in some individuals. Conduct a patch test before use.

Tea Tree Essential Oil

- Description: Tea tree oil has a medicinal and herbaceous scent, renowned for its antibacterial and antifungal properties.
- Common Uses: It is commonly used for skin issues and is an ingredient in natural insect repellents.
- Warnings: Tea tree oil is generally safe when used topically but may cause skin irritation in some individuals. Always conduct a patch test.

6

Cookie Recipes

Time to whip up something tasty with your favorite essential oils – and this time, you get to eat it! How exciting is that? Let's dive into the delicious world of yumminess!

6.1 Citrus Burst Cookies

Ingredients

- 2 cups all-purpose flour
- 1 cup unsalted butter, softened
- 1/2 cup powdered sugar
- 1 teaspoon vanilla extract
- 10 drops sweet orange essential oil

Instructions

1. Preheat the oven to 350°F (175°C).
2. In a mixing bowl, cream together the softened butter and powdered sugar until a smooth consistency is achieved.
3. Add the vanilla extract and 10 drops of sweet orange essential oil, mixing well.
4. Gradually incorporate the flour into the mixture, stirring until a dough forms.
5. Drop rounded spoonfuls of the dough onto a baking sheet.
6. Bake for 10-12 minutes or until the edges are lightly golden.
7. Allow the Citrus Burst Cookies to cool before serving. Enjoy the delightful citrus flavor!

Shopping List

- All-purpose flour
- Unsalted butter
- Powdered sugar
- Vanilla extract
- Sweet orange essential oil

Essential Oil Information

Sweet Orange Essential Oil

- Description: Sweet orange essential oil, derived from Citrus sinensis, imparts a bright and citrusy aroma. Known for its uplifting and energizing properties, it adds a burst of freshness to various culinary creations.
- Common Uses: Commonly used to uplift mood, promote relaxation,

and add a bright, citrusy aroma to blends in aromatherapy and homemade cleaning products.

- Warnings: Quality: Ensure the essential oil used is food-grade for culinary applications. Photosensitivity: Avoid exposure to direct sunlight after consuming, as citrus oils may cause photosensitivity.

6.2 Peppermint Chocolate Chip Cookies

Ingredients

- 2 1/4 cups all-purpose flour
- 1 cup unsalted butter, softened
- 3/4 cup granulated sugar
- 3/4 cup brown sugar, packed
- 2 large eggs
- 1 teaspoon vanilla extract
- 1/2 teaspoon baking soda
- 1/2 teaspoon salt
- 1 cup chocolate chips
- 5 drops peppermint essential oil

Instructions

1. Preheat the oven to 375°F (190°C).
2. In a large bowl, cream together softened butter, granulated sugar, and packed brown sugar until smooth.
3. Add eggs one at a time, beating well after each addition.
4. Stir in vanilla extract and 5 drops peppermint essential oil.
5. In a separate bowl, whisk together flour, baking soda, and salt.

6. Gradually add the dry ingredients to the wet ingredients, mixing until well combined.
7. Fold in chocolate chips.
8. Drop rounded tablespoons of dough onto baking sheets.
9. Bake for 9-11 minutes or until the edges are golden brown.
10. Allow the Peppermint Chocolate Chip Cookies to cool on the baking sheets for a few minutes before transferring to a wire rack. Enjoy the minty chocolate goodness!

Shopping List

- All-purpose flour
- Unsalted butter
- Granulated sugar
- Brown sugar
- Large eggs
- Vanilla extract
- Baking soda
- Salt
- Chocolate chips
- Peppermint essential oil

Essential Oil Information

Peppermint Essential Oil

- Description: Peppermint essential oil, derived from Mentha × piperita, offers a refreshing and minty aroma. Known for its invigorating properties, it adds a cool and lively flavor to culinary delights.
- Common Uses: Enhance recipes with a few drops for a delightful

minty twist. Add to hot chocolate or coffee for a minty flavor.

- Warnings: Ensure the essential oil used is food-grade for culinary applications. Use sparingly; peppermint oil is potent. Not for Internal Use when undiluted.

6.3 Lavender Shortbread Cookies

Ingredients

- 2 cups all-purpose flour
- 1 cup unsalted butter, softened
- 1/2 cup powdered sugar
- 1 teaspoon vanilla extract
- 1 tablespoon dried culinary lavender buds (finely chopped) (optional)
- 5 drops lavender essential oil

Instructions

1. Preheat the oven to 325°F (163°C).
2. In a bowl, cream together softened butter and powdered sugar until creamy.
3. Add vanilla extract, finely chopped lavender buds, and 5 drops of lavender essential oil, mixing well.
4. Gradually add the flour, mixing until a soft dough forms.
5. Roll the dough into a log shape, wrap in plastic wrap, and refrigerate for at least 1 hour.
6. Slice the chilled dough into rounds and place on a baking sheet.
7. Bake for 12-15 minutes or until the edges are lightly golden.
8. Let the Lavender Shortbread Cookies cool before serving.

Shopping List

- All-purpose flour
- Unsalted butter
- Powdered sugar
- Vanilla extract
- Dried culinary lavender buds (optional)
- Lavender essential oil

Essential Oil Information

Lavender Essential Oil

- Description: Lavender essential oil, extracted from Lavandula angustifolia, presents a sweet and floral aroma. Recognized for its calming properties, it adds a subtle and delightful flavor to culinary creations.
- Common Uses: Elevate recipes with a few drops for a floral touch. Tea Infusions: Add a drop to herbal teas for a hint of lavender flavor.
- Warnings: Quality: Ensure the essential oil used is food-grade for culinary applications. Quantity: Use sparingly; lavender oil is potent. Pregnancy: Consult with a healthcare professional before using lavender oil during pregnancy.

6.4 Lemon Poppy Seed Cookies

Ingredients

- 2 cups all-purpose flour
- 1 cup unsalted butter, softened
- 1/2 cup granulated sugar
- Zest of 2 lemons
- 2 tablespoons poppy seeds
- 1 teaspoon vanilla extract
- 8 drops lemon essential oil

Instructions

1. Preheat the oven to 350°F (175°C).
2. In a large bowl, cream together softened butter and granulated sugar until light and fluffy.
3. Add lemon zest, poppy seeds, vanilla extract, and 8 drops of lemon essential oil, mixing well.
4. Gradually add the flour, mixing until a dough forms.
5. Drop rounded spoonsful of dough onto a baking sheet.
6. Bake for 10-12 minutes or until the edges are golden.
7. Cool the Lemon Poppy Seed Cookies on a wire rack before serving. Enjoy the delightful citrus and poppy seed combination!

Shopping List

- All-purpose flour
- Unsalted butter
- Granulated sugar
- Lemons (for zest)

- Poppy seeds
- Vanilla extract
- Lemon essential oil

Essential Oil Information

Lemon Essential Oil

- Description: Lemon essential oil, extracted from Citrus limon, offers a bright and citrusy aroma. Known for its uplifting and refreshing properties, it adds a burst of citrus flavor to culinary delights.
- Common Uses: Cooking: Enhance recipes with a few drops for a zesty twist. Beverages: Add a drop to water or beverages for a hint of lemon flavor.
- Warnings: Quality: Ensure the essential oil used is food-grade for culinary applications. Photosensitivity: Avoid exposure to direct sunlight after consuming, as citrus oils may cause photosensitivity. Dilution: Use sparingly; lemon oil is potent.

6.5 Cinnamon Spice Snickerdoodle Cookies

Ingredients

- 2 3/4 cups all-purpose flour
- 1 cup unsalted butter, softened
- 1 1/2 cups granulated sugar
- 2 large eggs
- 1 teaspoon vanilla extract
- 1 teaspoon cream of tartar

- 1/2 teaspoon baking soda
- 1/4 teaspoon salt
- 8 drops cinnamon bark essential oil

Instructions

1. Preheat the oven to 375°F (190°C).
2. In a large bowl, cream together softened butter, granulated sugar, and eggs until smooth.
3. Add vanilla extract and 8 drops of cinnamon bark essential oil, mixing well.
4. In a separate bowl, whisk together flour, cream of tartar, baking soda, and salt.
5. Gradually add the dry ingredients to the wet ingredients, mixing until well combined.
6. Roll tablespoon-sized balls of dough in the cinnamon-sugar mixture.
7. Place the coated dough balls on a baking sheet, spacing them apart.
8. Bake for 8-10 minutes or until the edges are set.
9. Allow the Cinnamon Spice Snickerdoodles to cool on the baking sheet for a few minutes before transferring to a wire rack. Enjoy the warm and comforting flavor!

Shopping List

- All-purpose flour
- Unsalted butter
- Granulated sugar
- Eggs
- Vanilla extract
- Cream of tartar

- Baking soda
- Salt
- Cinnamon bark essential oil

Essential Oil Information

Cinnamon Bark Essential Oil

- Description: Cinnamon bark essential oil, derived from Cinnamo-mum verum, provides a warm and spicy aroma. Known for its comforting and invigorating properties, it adds a rich flavor to culinary creations.
- Common Uses: Elevate recipes with a few drops for a warm and aromatic twist. Hot Beverages: Add a drop to coffee or hot chocolate for a hint of cinnamon flavor.
- Warnings: Quality: Ensure the essential oil used is food-grade for culinary applications. Dilution: Use sparingly; cinnamon bark oil is potent. Do not ingest undiluted essential oil.

7

Body Scrub Recipes

Treat yourself to a mini spa day at home—because who says pampering is only for special occasions? Your skin will be singing 'thank you' for the VIP treatment! So, go ahead, let the good vibes flow, and give yourself the TLC you truly deserve!

7.1 Orange Chocolate Truffle Body Scrub

Ingredients

- 1 cup brown sugar
- 1/2 cup coconut oil
- 10 drops orange essential oil
- 1/4 cup cocoa powder

Instructions

1. In a bowl, mix 1 cup of brown sugar with 1/2 cup of coconut oil until well combined.
2. Add 10 drops of orange essential oil and 1/4 cup of cocoa powder to the sugar and oil mixture.
3. Stir the ingredients thoroughly to create a fragrant and luxurious Orange Chocolate Truffle Body Scrub.
4. Put the scrub into a small glass container with a lid.
5. Use the scrub in the shower by gently massaging it onto damp skin in circular motions.
6. Rinse off to reveal smooth and exfoliated skin. Enjoy the invigorating scent and the benefits of the natural ingredients in this amazing body scrub!

Shopping List

- Brown sugar
- Coconut oil
- Orange essential oil
- Cocoa powder
- Small glass container with lid

Essential Oil Information

Orange Essential Oil

- Description: Orange essential oil, extracted from Citrus sinensis, offers a sweet and citrusy aroma. Renowned for its uplifting and energizing properties, it adds a refreshing touch to skincare products.

- Common Uses: Body Scrub: Enhance body scrubs for a delightful citrus experience. Beauty Products: Incorporate into skincare routines for potential skin benefits.
- Warnings: Skin Sensitivity: Perform a patch test before applying directly to the skin. Photosensitivity: Avoid exposure to direct sunlight after applying to the skin, as citrus oils may cause photosensitivity. Dilution: Dilute properly before topical application.

7.2 Peppermint Patty Sugar Scrub

Ingredients

- 1 cup granulated sugar
- 1/2 cup almond oil
- 10 drops peppermint essential oil
- 1/4 cup cocoa powder

Instructions

1. In a bowl, combine 1 cup of granulated sugar with 1/2 cup of almond oil.
2. Mix in 10 drops of peppermint essential oil and 1/4 cup of cocoa powder to the sugar and oil mixture.
3. Stir the ingredients thoroughly to create a refreshing and invigorating Peppermint Patty Sugar Scrub.
4. Place the scrub in a small glass container with a lid.
5. Gently massage the scrub onto damp skin using circular motions, allowing the sugar to exfoliate and moisturize.
6. Rinse off with warm water to reveal smooth and rejuvenated

skin. Enjoy the delightful peppermint aroma and the pampering experience of this natural sugar scrub!

Shopping List

- Granulated sugar
- Almond oil
- Peppermint essential oil
- Cocoa powder
- Small glass container with a lid

Essential Oil Information

Peppermint Essential Oil

- Description: Peppermint essential oil, derived from Mentha × piperita, offers a cool and invigorating aroma. Known for its refreshing properties, it adds a revitalizing touch to skincare routines.
- Common Uses: Sugar Scrub: Enhance sugar scrubs for a refreshing and aromatic experience. Muscle Relief: Dilute and apply topically for a soothing massage on tired muscles.
- Warnings: Skin Sensitivity: Perform a patch test before applying directly to the skin. Avoid Eyes: Keep away from the eyes and mucous membranes. Not for Internal Use: Do not ingest undiluted essential oil.

7.3 Lemon Poppy Seed Exfoliating Scrub

Ingredients

- 1 cup white sugar
- 1/2 cup olive oil
- 15 drops lemon essential oil
- 1 tbsp poppy seeds

Instructions

1. In a mixing bowl, combine 1 cup of white sugar with 1/2 cup of olive oil.
2. Add 15 drops of lemon essential oil and 1 tbsp of poppy seeds to the sugar and oil mixture.
3. Stir the ingredients thoroughly to create a refreshing and gentle Lemon Poppy Seed Exfoliating Scrub.
4. Place the scrub into a small glass container with lid.
5. Use the scrub on damp skin, massaging it in circular motions for a gentle exfoliation.
6. Rinse off with warm water to reveal smooth and renewed skin. Enjoy the citrusy aroma and the rejuvenating benefits of this natural exfoliating scrub!

Shopping List

- White sugar
- Olive oil
- Lemon essential oil
- Poppy seeds
- Small glass container with lid

Essential Oil Information

Lemon Essential Oil

- Description: Lemon essential oil, extracted from Citrus limon, imparts a bright and citrusy aroma. Recognized for its uplifting and refreshing properties, it adds a burst of freshness to skincare routines.
- Common Uses: Exfoliating Scrub: Elevate scrubs for a revitalizing and aromatic experience. Cleaning: Add to homemade cleaning solutions for a fresh and clean scent.
- Warnings: Skin Sensitivity: Perform a patch test before applying directly to the skin. Photosensitivity: Avoid exposure to direct sunlight after applying to the skin, as citrus oils may cause photosensitivity. Dilution: Dilute properly before topical application.

7.4 Vanilla Lavender Bath Salts

Ingredients

- 1 cup Epsom salt
- 1/4 cup baking soda
- 10 drops vanilla essential oil
- 5 drops lavender essential oil

Instructions

1. In a mixing bowl, combine 1 cup of Epsom salt with 1/4 cup of baking soda.
2. Add 10 drops of vanilla essential oil and 5 drops of lavender essential oil to the salt and baking soda mixture.
3. Mix the ingredients thoroughly to create fragrant Vanilla Lavender Bath Salts.
4. Place the salts into a small glass container with a lid.
5. Add a few tablespoons of the bath salts to warm bathwater.
6. Enjoy a relaxing soak, allowing the soothing aroma of vanilla and lavender to create a tranquil bath experience.

Shopping List

- Epsom salt
- Baking soda
- Vanilla essential oil
- Lavender essential oil
- Small glass container with lid

Essential Oils Information

Vanilla Essential Oil

1. Description: Vanilla essential oil, derived from Vanilla planifolia, imparts a warm and sweet aroma. Known for its comforting properties, it adds a soothing touch to bath products.
2. Common Uses: Bath Salts: Enhance bath salts for a relaxing and aromatic experience. Skincare: Add to skincare products for a delightful fragrance.

3. Warnings: Quality: Ensure the essential oil used is high-quality and free from synthetic additives. Dilution: Dilute properly before topical application.

Lavender Essential Oil

- Description: Lavender essential oil, extracted from Lavandula angustifolia, presents a floral and calming aroma. Renowned for its relaxation properties, it adds a tranquil touch to bath rituals.
- Common Uses: Bath Salts: Combine with other oils for a well-rounded bath experience. Sleep Aid: Add to bedtime routines for potential calming effects.
- Warnings: Pregnancy: Consult with a healthcare professional before using lavender oil during pregnancy. Skin Sensitivity: Perform a patch test before applying directly to the skin.

7.5 Chocolate Mint Lip Scrub

Ingredients

- 1 tbsp brown sugar
- 1 tbsp coconut oil
- 1/2 tsp cocoa powder
- 5 drops peppermint essential oil

Instructions

1. In a small bowl, combine 1 tbsp of brown sugar with 1 tbsp of coconut oil.
2. Mix in 1/2 tsp of cocoa powder and add 5 drops of peppermint essential oil to the sugar and oil mixture.
3. Stir the ingredients thoroughly to create a delightful Chocolate Mint Lip Scrub.
4. Place the scrub in a small glass container with a lid.
5. Gently exfoliate your lips using the scrub, using small circular motions.
6. Rinse your lips with warm water to reveal soft and refreshed skin. Enjoy the invigorating aroma and the pampering benefits of this natural lip scrub!

Shopping List

- Brown sugar
- Coconut oil
- Cocoa powder
- Peppermint essential oil
- Small glass container with lid

Essential Oil Information

Peppermint Essential Oil

- Description: Peppermint essential oil, derived from Mentha × piperita, provides a cool and invigorating aroma. Known for its refreshing properties, it adds a rejuvenating touch to skincare products.

- Common Uses: Lip Scrub: Enhance lip scrubs for a refreshing and aromatic experience. Headache Relief: Dilute and apply topically for potential relief from headaches.
- Warnings: Skin Sensitivity: Perform a patch test before applying directly to the skin. Avoid Eyes: Keep away from the eyes and mucous membranes. Not for undiluted Internal Use: Do not ingest undiluted essential oil.

8

Bonus Recipes

Okay, get ready for a treat! Here are five bonus essential oil recipes to spice things up. Because why stop here when we can keep the fun rolling, right?

8.1 Relaxing Lavender Pillow Spray

Ingredients

- 2 oz distilled water
- 1 oz vodka or witch hazel
- 15 drops lavender essential oil

Instructions

1. Combine 2 oz of distilled water and 1 oz of vodka or witch hazel in a small glass spray bottle.
2. Add 15 drops of lavender essential oil to the mixture.
3. Shake the bottle well to ensure thorough mixing.

4. Spritz the resulting blend onto pillows before bedtime.

Shopping List

- Distilled water
- Vodka or witch hazel
- Lavender essential oil
- Small glass spray bottle

Essential Oil Information

Lavender Essential Oil

- Description: Lavender essential oil, extracted from the lavender plant, boasts a sweet, floral aroma known for its calming and soothing properties.
- Common Uses: Pillow Spray: Enhance sleep quality by incorporating into DIY sprays, like the Relaxing Lavender Pillow Spray. Bath Relaxation: Mix with a carrier oil for a calming bath experience.
- Warnings: Skin Sensitivity: Conduct a patch test before applying directly to the skin. Pregnancy: Consult with a healthcare professional before using lavender oil during pregnancy. Pets: Keep out of reach of pets, as certain essential oils may be harmful to them.

8.2 Cooling Peppermint Foot Soak

Ingredients

- 1/2 cup Epsom salt
- 1/4 cup baking soda
- 10 drops peppermint essential oil

Instructions

1. In a bowl, combine 1/2 cup Epsom salt and 1/4 cup baking soda.
2. Add 10 drops of peppermint essential oil to the dry mixture.
3. Stir the ingredients well to ensure an even distribution of the essential oil.
4. Place the foot soak into a small glass container with a lid.
5. Add the mixture to a warm foot bath.
6. Soak your feet and enjoy the cooling and invigorating sensation.

Shopping List

- Epsom salt
- Baking soda
- Peppermint essential oil
- Small glass container with lid

Essential Oil Information

Peppermint Essential Oil

- Description: Peppermint essential oil, extracted from the peppermint plant, carries a refreshing and minty aroma. It is known for its cooling properties and invigorating scent.

- Common Uses: Foot Soak: Add a few drops to foot soaks for a cooling and revitalizing experience. Muscle Relaxation: Dilute and massage onto muscles for a soothing effect.
- Warnings: Skin Sensitivity: Perform a patch test before applying directly to the skin. Avoid Eyes: Avoid contact with eyes; if contact occurs, rinse with plenty of water. Not for Internal Use: Do not ingest peppermint oil.

8.3 Rose Geranium Hair Conditioner

Ingredients

- 1 cup apple cider vinegar
- 10 drops rose geranium essential oil

Instructions

1. In a suitable container combine 1 cup of apple cider vinegar with 10 drops of rose geranium essential oil.
2. Mix the ingredients thoroughly to ensure even distribution of the essential oil.
3. Place the hair conditioner into a small glass container.
4. After shampooing, use the rose geranium hair conditioner as a final rinse for your hair.
5. Pour the mixture over your hair, ensuring it covers the strands.
6. Rinse your hair with water after applying the conditioner for a refreshing and fragrant finish.

Shopping List

- Apple cider vinegar
- Rose geranium essential oil
- Small glass container with lid

Essential Oil Information

Rose Geranium Essential Oil

- Description: Rose geranium essential oil, derived from the Pelargonium graveolens plant, exhibits a floral and sweet aroma reminiscent of roses. It is renowned for its balancing properties and appealing fragrance.
- Common Uses: Hair Care: Add to hair care products or create a hair conditioner for a pleasant scent and potential balancing effects. Skincare: Dilute and apply topically for potential skin benefits.
- Warnings: Skin Sensitivity: Perform a patch test before applying directly to the skin. Pregnancy: Consult with a healthcare professional before using rose geranium oil during pregnancy. Storage: Keep in a cool, dark place away from direct sunlight.

8.4 Orange Blossom Room Spray

Ingredients

- 2 oz distilled water
- 1 oz vodka or witch hazel
- 15 drops sweet orange essential oil

Instructions

1. In a small glass spray bottle, combine 2 oz of distilled water and 1 oz of vodka or witch hazel.
2. Add 15 drops of sweet orange essential oil to the mixture.
3. Shake the container well to ensure thorough mixing.
4. Use the Orange Blossom Room Spray as a refreshing spray in any room by gently misting the air.
5. Enjoy the uplifting and citrusy aroma that fills the space.

Shopping List

- Distilled water
- Vodka or witch hazel
- Sweet orange essential oil
- Small glass spray bottle

Essential Oil Information

Sweet Orange Essential Oil

- Description: Sweet orange essential oil, extracted from the peel of Citrus sinensis, emits a vibrant, citrusy aroma. Known for its uplifting properties, it adds a refreshing and energizing scent to various applications.
- Common Uses: Room Spray: Create an invigorating atmosphere by using in room sprays like the Orange Blossom Room Spray. Cleaning: Add to homemade cleaning solutions for a fresh scent.
- Warnings: Photosensitivity: Avoid exposure to direct sunlight after applying to the skin, as citrus oils may cause photosensitivity. Skin Sensitivity: Perform a patch test before applying directly to the

skin. Pets: Keep out of reach of pets, as certain essential oils may be harmful to them.

8.5 Bergamot and Chamomile Stress Relief Roller

Ingredients

- 2 tbsp sweet almond oil
- 10 drops bergamot essential oil
- 5 drops chamomile essential oil

Instructions

1. In a glass rollerball container, thoroughly mix 2 tbsp of sweet almond oil with 10 drops of bergamot essential oil and 5 drops of chamomile essential oil.
2. Apply the blend onto wrists and pulse points for stress relief.
3. Inhale the calming aroma and enjoy the soothing benefits throughout the day.

Shopping List

- Sweet almond oil
- Bergamot essential oil
- Chamomile essential oil
- Glass rollerball container

Essential Oil Information

Bergamot Essential Oil

- Description: Extracted from the Citrus bergamia fruit, bergamot essential oil offers a citrusy, sweet, and floral scent. Renowned for its uplifting and calming properties, it adds a refreshing touch to various applications.
- Common Uses: Stress Relief: Inhale the aroma or apply topically for stress reduction. Skincare: Dilute and apply to promote healthy-looking skin.
- Warnings: Photosensitivity: Avoid exposure to direct sunlight after applying to the skin, as citrus oils may cause photosensitivity. Skin Sensitivity: Perform a patch test before applying directly to the skin. Pregnancy: Consult with a healthcare professional before using bergamot oil during pregnancy.

Chamomile Essential Oil

- Description: Derived from the Matricaria chamomilla plant, chamomile essential oil has a sweet, herbaceous aroma known for its calming and soothing qualities.
- Common Uses: Relaxation: Inhale or apply for relaxation and emotional well-being. Sleep Aid: Diffuse or apply before bedtime to promote restful sleep. Skincare: Dilute and use in skincare routines for potential skin benefits.
- Warnings: Allergies: Avoid if allergic to plants in the Asteraceae family. Pregnancy: Consult with a healthcare professional before using chamomile oil during pregnancy.

9

Conclusion

I had such a great time making this recipe book! Thanks so much for purchasing it. By this point in the book, you've probably had a blast making some of these essential oil recipes. If not, now's the time to pick a couple and go for it! You won't be disappointed!

If you found this book helpful, I'd really appreciate it if you would leave a favorable review on Amazon. Thank you!

10

Essential Oils and Recipes Index

Peppermint essential oil

Lavender Mint Soap

Rosemary and Peppermint Energizing Soap

Peppermint Cocoa Lip Balm

Lavender Mint Lip Balm

Coconut Lime Lip Balm

Basic Bug Spray

Peppermint Chocolate Chip Cookies

Peppermint Patty Sugar Scrub

Chocolate Mint Lip Scrub

Cooling Peppermint Foot Soak

Rose geranium essential oil

Rose Geranium Hair Conditioner

Rosemary essential oil

Rosemary and Peppermint Energizing Soap

Rosemary Citrus Tick Repellent

Sweet orange essential oil

Citrus Burst Cookies

Orange Blossom Room Spray

Tea tree essential oil

Tea Tree & Eucalyptus Antibacterial Soap

Eucalyptus and Tea Tree Anti-Mosquito Spray

Vanilla essential oil

Vanilla Honey Lip Balm

Vanilla Lavender Bath Salts

11

References

OpenAI. (2022). ChatGPT: A powerful language model by OpenAI. https://openai.com/chatgpt